Living Healthy:
A Practical Guide to Your Optimal Health

Copyright © 2015 by UImpact Publishing
All Rights Reserved

1.Health & Fitness 2. Healthy Living
ISBN-10: 0692571914 / ISBN-13: 978-0692571910

Michelle Brown Stephenson,
BSN, MLS, MS, CHES
RN, Health Educator

Health Options & Alternatives

To my husband Carl Edward Stephenson, it is truly my privilege to be your life partner. Thank you for your unconditional love and friendship. To my children Kyrell Janae' & Kyra Janelle; it is an honor to watch you grow and blossom into beautiful young ladies. With all my love.

Why I Wrote This Book:

Individuals want and need reliable health information that is communicated in everyday language. It is my endeavor to elevate that perceived knowledge deficit where health education is concerned. My desire is for every person to have the understanding and ability to converse intelligently with their healthcare team when the situation arises. To that end; the general public has to begin the conversation on their role and responsibility in controlling their own personal health. Healthy does not just happen; it is a disciplined lifestyle that yields it.

I sincerely believe that if people have tangible basic information that they can grasp, they can make better choices that lead to significant improvements in their quality of life. I choose to dedicate my professional career to assisting others to empowerment. I choose to teach those who desire to learn health. I choose to listen, inspire learning, and communicate health knowledge in a humble and giving manner.

THE FOUNDATIONAL BALANCE MODEL

I do commend and applaud you for taking the time and exerting the effort to learn more of how to take care of your health. To have the opportunity to serve as your facilitating guide through this transition is an extraordinary honor and profound responsibility. I do not enter into this partnership with you lightly and I am committed to ensuring you have the tools you need to make this happen. The ultimate goal/reason for this small book is to facilitate understanding. I want to give you a working knowledge of the six components which in proper balance act as catalysts to living healthy.

It is a well-known fact that most of the general population tend to be confused when it comes to the basics of fostering a healthy lifestyle. The media consistently reports the next great fad. Evidenced based practice is not consistently portrayed in the best light. In such, the foundational balance model offers the general public a simple focus point that is evidence- based modifiable behaviors, the individual can control. This book will not only provide you with a working model that can be implemented in your daily regimen, but can be shared with your family and friends.

Our health care system has been focused on sickness and disease. From acute illness to chronic diseases, infectious diseases to degenerative diseases - we know what contributes to illness. We have developed some treatment modalities (surgery, radiation, chemotherapy etc...) for chronic symptoms and even a few cures for some chronic conditions. Heart disease, cancer, stroke, respiratory diseases, high blood pressure, diabetes and excessive alcohol consumption are just a few conditions that we know can wreak havoc on our physical, emotional and financial health. This book will help you to make the transition and start the conversation to change.

We need a different focus in healthcare delivery, one that contributes to wellness. Healthcare providers have shifted the focus, and now understand that PREVENTION is the key! Research has shown that diet, exercise, and healthy lifestyle behaviors along with preventive health screenings contribute to the increase in the quality and quantity of an individual's life. The Center for Disease Control (CDC) says "Every day, people confront situations that involve life-changing decisions about their health. These decisions are made in places such as grocery and drug stores, workplaces, playgrounds, doctors' offices, clinics and hospitals, and around the kitchen table. Obtaining, communicating, processing, and understanding health information and services are essential steps in making appropriate health decisions."

Research from The State of Aging and Health in America reported that nearly 9 of 10 adults have trouble using the everyday health information that is routinely available in our health care facilities, retail outlets, media, and communities. Without clear information and an understanding of the information's importance, people are more likely to skip necessary medical tests, end up in the emergency room more often, and have a harder time managing chronic diseases such as diabetes or high blood pressure.

HOPE for the hopeless:

I am really honored and happy that you have chosen to meet me here to discuss and/or bring back to your remembrance some healthy facts that you have known all your life. Why am I so passionate about this issue of health? Well, let me briefly tell you a small portion of my story. Growing up in my home, I just assumed that every other household was just like mine. I assumed everyone drank homemade fruit juice in the morning and homemade vegetable juice in the evenings. I believed what my parents told me which was that every child needed their rainbow of foods to ensure they were adequately prepared for the day. It was not until I reached high school that I realized that not every student brought their lunch, and their lunches didn't consist of any of the hummus and avocado sandwiches I had grown to love. The other kids didn't bring a small green thermos full of okra with crackers. It was a rude awakening for me when some of the other children started to notice that my lunches were totally different from the "normal" sandwich chips and a drink. I was even called hurtful names by a few. So as you can imagine when I completed high school and went off to college, I determined that I would change what I knew about nutrition and fit/blend in with the main stream.

I started to consume all sorts of fast foods. I relinquished my fruits and veggies for lunch meat with cheese with a side of chips. Over time I began to notice various changes in my physical appearance, my skin, hair, nails, eyes and teeth. All of my dietary changes had detrimental effects on my body.

I have experienced my fair share of health issues. I myself am a cancer survivor. I am the mom of two beautiful blessings. Both were born prematurely. The first was born at 6 months' gestation at 1lb 11oz. The second was born at 8 months' gestation. Both my parents sustained strokes later in life. My husband has experienced a life changing stroke as well. So I think I speak from an inside view of what health or the lack thereof can feel like. With so many issues at different times and stages all happening in a well-choreographed dance called life, I choose to understand what health is and inspire others to do the same. I came to a point in my life where the light came on very bright.

It finally dawned on me that when I consumed what my parents had instilled in me at an early age about health and nutrition my body never experienced symptoms of sickness. So I made a conscious choice to re-visited the concepts that alternative and complementary medicine are built upon. I have grouped them together in what I call the Foundational Balance Model. I know that sounds so clinical in nature but that is my educational background.

Most individuals make food decisions based on taste, but our bodies make decisions based on nutrition. There are just a few essential items the body requires to carry out metabolic processes and activities of daily living. When we are attempting to increase our risk to become healthy, we must look at what the body needs to run at its optimal strength. The goal here is for you to grasp the concept of balance, so that you understand what and how you along with the decisions you make control your health. Have you heard of RISK FACTORS? It is said that risk factors are conditions or habits that make a person more likely to develop a disease. They can also increase the chances that an existing disease will get worse. You need to know how to increase your risk factors for health!

The Resolution:

I submit to you, the reader of this book, that you CAN increase your "RISK" for or toward healthy. Let us get a mental image of a number line.

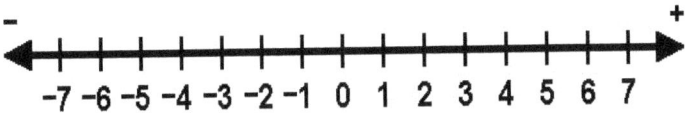

The number line can stretch for quite a while in both directions. In the middle is zero and on either side are the negative and the positive numbers. Let's view the negative numbers as the illness/disease continuum and the positive numbers as the healthy portion of the continuum. These two poles are exact opposites. With that being said; I submit to you that you CAN increase your risk of becoming your optimal healthy self.

LET'S DEFINE:
Disease and
Being Healthy

Disease and Healthy:

Let's look at a two terms that will allow us to come together and understand just what we are all working so hard to achieve. These two terms are the opposite poles we just spoke about. I submit that we live our lives on a continuum between these two poles. We make choices that move us along this continuum. It's like that huge number line with each individual person occupying the zero in the middle of the number line.

There is a positive end (healthy) and a negative end (disease). The daily choices we make impact our end result either positively or on the converse negatively. What are some behaviors we continue to engage in that have negative outcomes? Smoking, excessive drinking, sedentary lifestyles, overeating, consuming fast foods on a regular basis, choosing not to eat fruits and vegetables, choosing not to drink water, over using legal pharmaceuticals, consuming illegal substances, and choosing to forgo sleep, etc. These actions over time all contribute to negative moves along that continuum.

Our bodies are magnificent yet delicate. The body was designed to fluctuate on the imaginary number line between -1 and +1. We will see and feel drastic symptoms when we continually add in more negatives. Over time, the score; our score of pluses and minuses add up and we see the manifestation of our choices in our physical bodies. So let us fully understand these two terms. The first term is disease. Here is a working definition, granted it's crude to say the least but it will paint a picture or give you a vivid image to hold in your mind.

Disease – Any illness that affects a person, a condition that prevents the body or mind from working normally (properly). If you dissect the word, dis/ease, a body that is not at ease. Some examples include but are not limited to: Heart Disease, Stroke, Cancer, Diabetes Mellitus, Hypertension, Obesity, Constipation, Skin Diseases, Arthritis, Respiratory Diseases, Oral Conditions. The second of the two terms is healthy. This term is not a one-time situation or even a single decision. It is not reserved only for the young or the people under a certain age. Here is a working definition.

Healthy – The sum total of personal decisions/choices which an individual has control over, and participates in on a regular basis, that contribute positively to their quality and quantity of life. What are some behaviors we continue to participate in that positively affect us? Active lifestyles with plenty of age appropriate exercise, choosing to regularly eat well-balanced meals, choosing to drink adequate amounts of water daily, choosing to rest and relax with proper sleep patterns, choosing to maintain gender and ethnicity appropriate body weight, choosing to monitor hereditary risk factors and be an active participant in their own healthcare, etc.

Our Actions Have Enormous Consequences!

The solution is so profound, yet so simple. It starts and ends with the choices we make and expands exponentially. Now, what if we turn our thoughts to that Foundational Balance Model? Take a look at the image below, we will break it down in sections and briefly discuss each component.

There are six components that are essential. As the given name implies there is a delicate balance that must be adhered to. If you weigh in more on one portion of the model than another, the equilibrium will be offset and imbalance/instability occurs.

The six are as follows:

- Water
- Nutrition
- Proper Breathing
- Adequate Elimination
- Sleep
- Exercise.

Give me just a short bit of your time and we can discuss each of the components and a few tips to help you along the way.

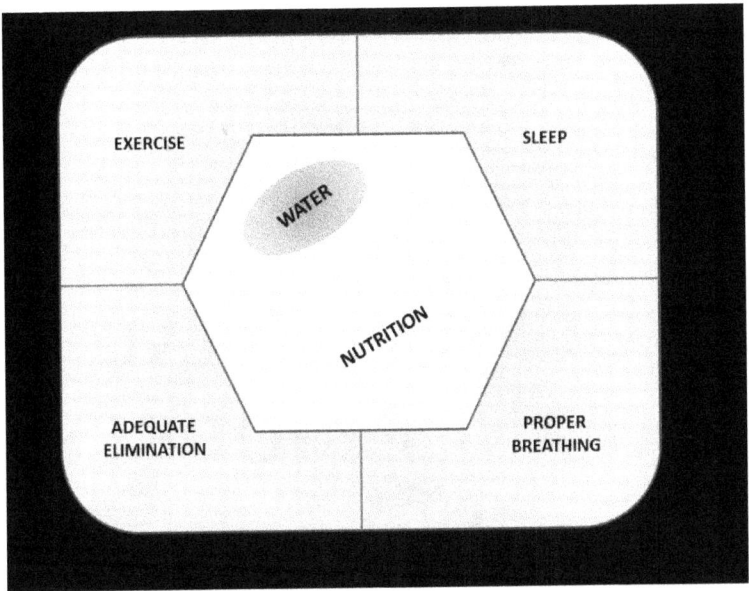

THE FOUNDATIONAL BALANCE MODEL: Water

There are many benefits that come along with drinking water: Regulates body temperature, lubricates & cushions the joints, lessens the burden on the kidneys & liver by flushing out waste products. Water carries nutrients & oxygen to cells, helps dissolve minerals & other nutrients to make them accessible to the body and helps prevent constipation. Water protects body organs and tissues (ie spinal cord & other sensitive tissues) and Moistens tissues such as those in the mouth, eyes, nose, and ears. Water disposes of waste through urination, perspiration and bowel movements.

Water is the body's principal chemical component & makes up approx. 60% of your body weight. Every system in the body depends on water. Lack of water can lead to dehydration, a condition that occurs when you do not have enough water in the body to carry out normal functions. The Institute of Medicine determined that adequate intake for a man is roughly 3 liters or 13 cups of total beverages per day. The adequate intake for women is roughly 22 liters or 9 cups of total beverages per day. In 2004 the Food & Nutrition Board released new dietary reference intakes for water. It is recommended that men consume 3.7 liters and women consume 2.7 liters.

Here is what I explain to any class or workshop I facilitate concerning water intake. For every hour that you are awake – Drink 1 -8oz glass/cup/container. Now do understand this is provided your physician has not placed you on fluid restriction. The Center for Disease Control (CDC) & American Council of Exercise state that the body can only process 17 to 20 oz of water per drinking cycle. What does this mean in layman's terms? I know you have always heard that you should consume 64 oz of water per day. Well that is very true, however; your body cannot process that much water at any given time. You must space it out over time throughout the day. Take home message: If you stop at the convenience store and buy a 32 oz bottle of water, you can only drink a portion of it right away. Your body can only handle 20 oz (maximum) at any given time. The rest of the water from that 32 oz bottle (12 oz) is sending you to the restroom (over working your kidneys) or third spacing (causing swelling in your arms legs hands and feet).

THE FOUNDATIONAL BALANCE MODEL:
Nutrition

It's pleasing to the palate and attractive to the eye. We must consume a nutritional rainbow in order to have a diet that is full of variety. The six essential nutrients required by the human body include carbohydrates, protein, fat, vitamins, minerals and water. Without these vital components our cells are not able to divide and multiply. When we consume a variety of different colors of fruits and vegetables we give our bodies the necessary ingredients to allow basic metabolic processes to occur.

Benefits of adding a rainbow (variety) to your diet as published by the MayoClinic:

- Eating a diet rich in vegetables and fruits as part of an overall healthy diet may reduce risk for heart disease, including heart attack and stroke and may protect against certain types of cancers.
- Eating vegetables and fruits rich in potassium as part of an overall healthy diet may lower blood pressure, may also reduce the risk of developing kidney stones, and help to decrease bone loss.
- Eating foods such as fruits and vegetables that are lower in calories per cup, instead of some other

higher-calorie food may be useful in helping to lower calorie intake.

- Diets rich in foods containing fiber, such as some vegetables and fruits, may reduce the risk of heart disease, obesity, and type 2 diabetes.
- Increase the vitamins and minerals you intake by adding a rainbow of colors as you choose the fruits and vegetables you enjoy daily and you will also increase the health benefit.

As you lower and eventually control your disease process through and because of your consistent dietary changes, you decrease the risk of heart disease, stroke, cancer, respiratory diseases, and high blood pressure. Understand that for taste purposes, most people inter-mingle certain fruits and veggies as in salads and on sandwiches.

Here are a few "did you know's" to facilitate your transformation to a new and better you:

- Fruits are cleansers and they sweep the colon. Just remember a quick rule of thumb - Fruits have seeds. Fruits are excellent for breakfast and great for a snack.

- Vegetables are builders they boost the immune system. Just remember a quick rule of thumb - Vegetables do not have seeds and they are excellent for lunch & dinner, great as healthy, hearty snacks.

How to make a fruit salad:

Choose a rainbow: look for various colors 5-7 or more if you like. I enjoy different shapes and it makes the presentation later very interesting, so I dice some small squares and cut others in a longer strips. Be creative and make it fun.

Here are a few to get you started:

- Apple
- Watermelon
- Cantaloupe
- Peach
- Plum
- Nectarine
- Honey Dew

- Pineapple
- Strawberry
- Grapes (white, black, red, green)
- Blueberries
- Kiwi
- Raspberries
- Blackberries
- Pears
- Oranges
- Tangerines

Place your 5 to 7 fruits in a bowl as your cut/slice/dice/cube them. You have now completed making a fruit salad! Now for the finishing touch to keep them looking pleasing to the eye add a couple of sprinkles of lemon juice (fresh or out of the bottle you buy from the grocery store). We do not want your masterpiece to turn brown. If you forget to add the lemon juice, some fruits will turn brown.

How to make a vegetable salad:

First off you must choose the type of foundation you would like. The foundation can be any type of lettuce and there is a variety to pick from: iceberg, romaine, kale, spring mix, spinach, etc. Next you add the vegetables and or fruits you want on top such as cucumber tomato mushroom carrots onion (there are several types so experiment and find out which suit you) celery quinoa radish tri colored bell pepper just to name a few. Please know this salad is fresh so it will start to wilt in a few days. You can add a sprinkle of lemon to the cut toppings to keep them from turning brown.

Remember the colors of the fruits and vegetable have different nutritional properties that the body requires so variety is the key. Here is an image from Physicians Committee for Responsible Medicine to assist you in understanding.

The Nutrition Rainbow

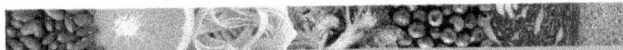

Tips From The Cancer Project: *The more naturally colorful your meal is, the more likely it is to have an abundance of cancer-fighting nutrients. Pigments that give fruits and vegetables their bright colors represent a variety of protective compounds. The chart below shows the cancer-fighting and immune-boosting power of different-hued foods.*

Colors	Foods	Colorful Protective Substances and Possible Actions
Red	Tomatoes and tomato products, watermelon, guava	Lycopene: antioxidant; cuts prostate cancer risk
Orange	Carrots, yams, sweet potatoes, mangos, pumpkins	Beta-carotene: supports immune system; powerful antioxidant
Yellow-orange	Oranges, lemons, grapefruits, papayas, peaches	Vitamin C, flavonoids: inhibit tumor cell growth, detoxify harmful substances
Green	Spinach, kale, collards, and other greens	Folate: builds healthy cells and genetic material
Green-white	Broccoli, Brussels sprouts, cabbage, cauliflower	Indoles, lutein: eliminate excess estrogen and carcinogens
White-green	Garlic, onions, chives, asparagus	Allyl sulfides: destroy cancer cells, reduce cell division, support immune systems
Blue	Blueberries, purple grapes, plums	Anthocyanins: destroy free radicals
Red-purple	Grapes, berries, plums	Resveratrol: may decrease estrogen production
Brown	Whole grains, legumes	Fiber: carcinogen removal

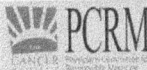

PCRM

5100 Wisconsin Avenue, NW, Suite 400 • Washington, DC 20016
202-244-5038 • www.CancerProject.org

The Cancer Project, a division of Physicians Committee for Responsible Medicine, is dedicated to advancing cancer prevention and survival through nutrition education and research.

THE
FOUNDATIONAL
BALANCE MODEL:
Adequate Elimination

When the body has extracted all of the useful vitamins and minerals from our items we intake then the leftovers are considered waste products. The body must excrete those somehow. Ear wax, feces, urine, perspiration, nasal discharge, various gases etc...

For every meal that you consume, you should have a bowel movement. It's a one for one return. The body must process what goes in. Digestion ensures that the vital nutrients are removed. The items that are not used will be left as waste.

Constipation is the results of consuming more meals than you have adequate elimination to match. Also, a bit of information you should be aware of, the body will attempt to compensate for all that you ingest. The body can only compensate for so long. This is when we start to see manifestation of illness and disease, when the body can no longer compensate for your actions. Long story short, if you consume 3-6 meals per day but you only eliminate once or twice a day, your body must store that waste somewhere. Now let's think about this, if you consume 3-6 meals per day but you only eliminate weekly or maybe even every two weeks. We are overworking the system and breakdown/wipeout is only a matter of time. For those that are interested please take a look online for a bowel scale. The information may just save your life.

Here is an image from www.healthworks.my I show it in classes and workshops to facilitate understanding and potentially start the dialogue about stool.

How Well Do You Know Your Poop?

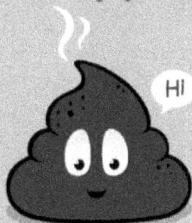

When you poop, the little brown blob in your toilet bowl is what's left of the food after your body has absorbed all the nutrients it needs from it.

Pooping is vital to your health as it's your body's natural way of expelling the waste that it doesn't need. That's why how you poop looks and smells can also give clues to what's going on inside your body.

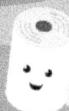

Textures of poop

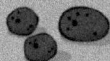

Separate hard lumps, like nuts
You're lacking fibre and fluids. Drink more water and chomp on some fruits and veggies.

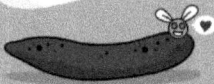

Sausage-shaped but lumpy
Not as serious as separate hard lumps, but you need to load up on fluids and fibre.

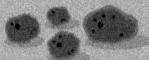

Sausage-shaped but with cracks on surface
This is normal, but the cracks mean you could still up your intake of water.

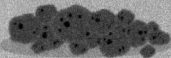

Sausage-shaped, smooth and soft
Optimal poop! You're doing fine!

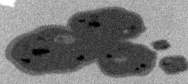

Soft blobs with clear-cut edges
Not too bad. Pretty normal if you're pooping multiple times a day.

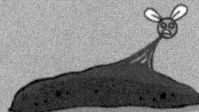

Fluffy pieces with ragged edges, a mushy stool
You're on the edge of normal. This type of poop is on its way to becoming diarrhoea.

Watery, no solid pieces, all liquid
You're having diarrhoea! This is probably caused by some sort of infection and diarrhoea is your body's way of cleaning it out. Make sure you drink lots of liquids to replace the liquids lost otherwise you might find yourself dehydrated!

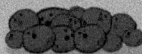

Soft and sticks to the side of the toilet bowl
Presence of too much oil, which could mean that your body isn't absorbing the fats properly. Diseases like chronic pancreatitis prevent your body from properly absorbing fat.

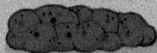

Shades of poop

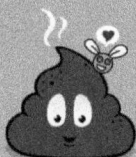

Brown: You're fine. Poop is naturally brown due to the bile produced in your liver.

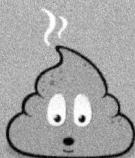

Green: Food may be moving through your large intestine too quickly. Or you could have eaten lots of green leafy veggies, or green food colouring.

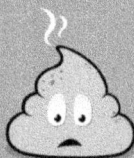

Yellow: Greasy, foul-smelling yellow poop indicates excess fat, which could be due to a malabsorption disorder like celiac disease.

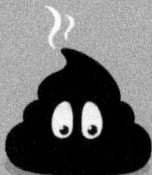

Black: It could mean that you're bleeding internally due to ulcer or cancer. Some vitamins containing iron or bismuth subsalicylate could cause black poop too. Pay attention if it's sticky, and see a doc if you're worried.

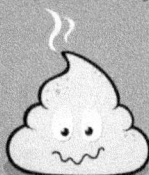

Light-coloured, white, or clay-coloured: If it's not what you're normally seeing, it could mean a bile duct obstruction. Some meds could cause this too. See a doc.

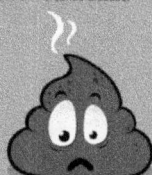

Blood-stained or Red: Blood in your poop could be a symptom of cancer. Always see a doc right away if you find blood in your stool.

Quick facts about poop

- The food you eat usually takes 1- 3 days from the time you eat it till it ends up in your poop.
- Poop is made up of undigested food, bacteria, mucus, and dead cells, that's why it smells.
- Healthy poop sinks slowly.

How often should you poop?

On average, people go once or twice a day, but some may go more and some may go less. According to doctors, there's no normal frequency, so as long as you're comfy, you're fine.

How to keep your poop healthy?

- Eat a diet high in fibre (20 – 25g), lots of water, regular exercise.
- If you're having trouble pooping (constipation), dietary fibre can help make the passage smoother.
- Proper hydration helps ensure your colon is slippery enough for the poop to move through.

When to see a doctor?

The first time you see anything out of the ordinary in your poop, don't panic yet. See if it happens again. If symptoms persist, then go talk to a doctor. Pay attention to what your body is telling you, and whenever you feel uneasy, it's time to go to a doctor.

THE FOUNDATIONAL BALANCE MODEL:
Proper Breathing

We take for granted that something so vital is done correctly, our bodies will compensate for as long as it can, but in the end; we lose if we are not breathing correctly. For a simple analogy, just think of your lungs as balloons. When you are not filling these vital balloons with air you leave them open and susceptible to fluid bacteria and mucous.

So how should we breathe? I'm glad you asked. We should take deep breaths every single time we inhale. It should go like this cute little jingle we teach our children: Smell the roses (this is the inhale) and blow out the candles on the cake (this is the exhale). Now we should utilize our noses for the entire process but when we are teaching the kids they must have a visual to follow, so we use our mouths for the exhale. Now as adults we should be able to do the process with our noses unless there is some obstruction/congestion going on in the respiratory track.

Everyone stand up PLEASE!, time to practice. I know you are reading this, but try and visualize this. Smell the roses (deeply) now hold, and then blow out the candles (pursed lips) this is proper breathing. It does not have to be done with the lips and mouth; it can flow out through the nose, but it must be deep and very intentional.

THE FOUNDATIONAL BALANCE MODEL: Sleep

Sleep is often one of the first things to go when people feel pressed for time. Many view sleep as a luxury and think that the benefits of limiting the hours they spend asleep outweigh the costs. People often overlook the potential long-term health consequences of insufficient sleep, and the impact that health problems can ultimately have on one's time and productivity.

Many of the costs of poor sleep go unnoticed. Medical conditions, such as obesity, diabetes, and cardiovascular disease, develop over long periods of time and result from a number of factors, such as genetics, poor nutrition, and lack of exercise. Insufficient sleep has also been linked to these and other health problems, and is considered an important risk factor. Although scientists have just begun to identify the connections between insufficient sleep and disease, most experts have concluded that getting enough high-quality sleep may be as important to health and well-being as nutrition and exercise. Numerous studies have found that insufficient sleep increases a person's risk of developing serious medical conditions, including obesity, diabetes, and cardiovascular disease. Not surprisingly, these potential adverse health effects can add up to increased health care costs and decreased productivity. More importantly, insufficient sleep can ultimately affect life expectancy and day-to-day well-being

Sleep, like nutrition and physical activity, is a critical determinant of health and well-being. Sleep loss and untreated sleep disorders influence basic patterns of behavior that negatively affect family health and interpersonal relationships. Adequate sleep is necessary to fight off infection, support the metabolism of sugar to prevent diabetes, perform well in school and work effectively and safely. Sleep timing and duration affect a number of endocrine, metabolic, and neurological functions that are critical to the maintenance of individual health. Fatigue and sleepiness can reduce productivity and increase the chance for mishaps such as medical errors and motor vehicle or industrial accidents.

While getting adequate sleeping alone is no guarantee of good health, it does help to maintain many vital functions. One of the most important of these functions may be to provide cells and tissues with the opportunity to recover from the wear and tear of daily life. Major restorative functions in the body such as tissue repair, muscle growth, and protein synthesis occur almost exclusively during sleep. Lack of adequate sleep over time has been associated with a shortened lifespan. Sleep and mood are closely connected; poor or inadequate sleep can cause irritability and stress, while healthy sleep can enhance well-being. Chronic insomnia may increase the risk of developing a mood disorder, such as anxiety or depression. Inadequate sleep appears to affect the brain's ability to consolidate both factual information and procedural memories about how to do various physical tasks as seen in studies by the Sleep Foundation. Can we agree that we need rest for rejuvenation??!!

THE
FOUNDATIONAL
BALANCE MODEL:
Exercise

In order to attain and maintain our physical mobility, flexibility, and agility we must actively participate in some type of exercise. Exercise controls weight, it combats health conditions and diseases, it improves mood, it boosts energy, and promotes better sleep. Calisthenics is loosely defined as a form of exercise consisting of a variety of exercises, often rhythmical, movements, generally without using equipment or apparatus. They are intended to increase body strength and flexibility with movements such as bending, jumping, swinging, twisting or kicking, using only one's body weight for resistance. There are many benefits to physical activity/exercise.

The benefits of calisthenics exercise are as follows:
- enable enormous strength and flexibility
- Increased cardio-respiratory endurance, muscle endurance, core strength, & endurance
- less likely to cause muscle or joint injuries which are so common in weight training
- can be performed anywhere therefore, no excuse for skipping workout

- with proper diet a good way to achieve a healthier, stronger, and more flexible body
- great form of exercise for beginners to advanced fitness enthusiasts.
- use your own body strength

There are other forms of exercise that may better suit your fancy such as walking, riding a bike or even weight lifting. Just make sure you are an active participant and you are doing both aerobic and anaerobic exercise. This will keep the body in balance.

How does one pebble dropped into a pond make so many waves? It's called the ripple effect. I submit this mini book as my humble offering to our Nation at large. My endeavor is to give responsibility and control back to the individual. By giving a starting point and promoting understanding, one person can assist many to change small behaviors that make huge differences. As you become aware of beneficial things you should share the knowledge so that others can make informed decisions. Please spread the word, tell your family, friends' and acquaintances', we can increase our RISK for and toward healthy. It's a way of living and not a single momentary choice

"A wise man should consider that health is the greatest of human blessing"

-Hippocrates

"There is only one good: Knowledge and one evil: Ignorance."

-Socrates

Michelle Brown Stephenson,
BSN, MLS, MS, CHES

Professional bio:

Simply known as "The Nurse", Michelle is a knowledgeable professional with years of practical experience. For more than 20 years she has provided valuable insight, interpretation and guidance to organizations, associations and individuals. She has a sixth sense when it comes to navigating her patients and clients through the maze of the available health care options, understanding health diagnoses & concerns, de-mystifying medical jargon. Michelle provides evidence based proven modalities and treatments that allow her patients and clients to play an active and integral role in their healthcare team. Her education credentials resemble alphabet soup and she is currently pursuing a Doctorate in Public Health.

When it comes to her professional philosophy, she believes, "I am dedicated to empowering others in their pursuit of health and healthy living. My desire and goal is to serve others by listening, inspiring, and educating individuals not only about health but about *their* health. My goal is to help others establish a legacy of health".

My desire and goal is to serve others by listening, inspiring, and educating individuals not only about health but about *their* health. My goal is to help others establish a legacy of health".

Personal Bio:

Born the eldest of two children to Sherman and Helen Brown in Chicago, IL. Michelle's secular education consists of an Associates of Arts, a Bachelor of Science in Nursing, and dual Masters Degrees in Health Education and Library Science. She is currently pursuing a Doctorate degree in Public Health.

Her secular employment has three components: Registered Nurse and Health Educator for the United States Public Health Service Commissioned Corps currently stationed at the Federal Bureau of Prisons.

Michelle accepted Jesus Christ into her life at the age of twelve. She was an active member of Cornerstone Baptist Church of Arlington, TX since

1988. Michelle lovingly and willingly surrendered her will to the Father in 1996. In 2002, she transitioned her membership to Higher Praise Family Church. Michelle was ordained as a deaconess in March 2012 and ordained as an elder in March 2013. She currently serves in the following ministries: Divine Health (Medical Ministry Leader), Women's Small Group Bible Study (Teacher/Facilitator), and Cultivating the Call (Facilitator/Instructor).

In 1997, she accepted God's plan and purpose for her life. Health Options and Alternatives, Inc. was founded from that call. Health Options & Alternatives is a non-profit organization whose purpose is to assist other to empowerment through health education. 3 John 2 states "Beloved, I pray that you may prosper in every way and [that your body] may keep well, even as [I know] your soul keeps well and prospers". (Amplified)

Michelle has been happily married to Carl E. Stephenson for twenty years. God is richly blessing and bringing increase in their union. They have two beautiful daughters (Kyrell & Kyra). Her favorite scripture is Proverbs 4:7, "The beginning of Wisdom is: get Wisdom (skillful and godly Wisdom)! [For skillful and godly Wisdom is the principal thing.] And with all you have gotten, get understanding (discernment, comprehension, and interpretation)". (Amplified)

About Health Options & Alternatives

Health Options & Alternatives (HOA) provides educational programs and services on developing a healthy lifestyle, nutrition, and avenues of alternative health care options.

The HOA teams are knowledgeable professionals with years of practical health care experience who provide valuable insight and interpretive guidance in helping organizations, associations and individuals navigate through the maze of the available health care options. Taking care of your health is of the utmost importance to us.

Have you ever wanted information on health related topics?

Have you or your loved one needed medical definitions, explanations, and current treatments?

HOA exists to assist you in understanding your health concerns. We provide evidence based, proven modalities and treatments.

Our Mission & Vision

HOA's threefold mission is:

- To be a health education and information resource complex, serving consumers and providers alike, designed to facilitate healthy lifestyles.
- To stand as a visible commitment of strategic alliances that empower our community as it seeks to enhance the quality of lives, through a variety of services that assist in obtaining and maintaining optimal health
- To provide a critical link in the network of multidisciplinary health resources in the Tarrant County area.

HOA's vision is threefold:

- To aid the client in increasing their knowledge foundation where health is concerned.
- To provide health education and information in a user friendly format, in a timely manner.
- To support the client through the stages of healthy behavior modification.

Our Commitment to Quality

- Health Options & Alternatives chooses to dedicate itself to assisting others to empowerment through education.
- Assisting those who desire to learn health; we choose to listen, inspire learning and communicate knowledge in a humble and giving manner.
- We pledge to facilitate innovative learning experiences designed to meet the needs of our clients.

Our Core Values

- Healthy is a way of living, not a single momentary choice.
- Facilitating healthy lifestyles through education and thus empowerment of the general public by providing a variety of services that assist in obtaining and maintaining optimal health.

Our Services:

✓ Health Care Summits

- ✓ Individual Assessments

- ✓ Online Library

- ✓ Onsite Training

- ✓ Certifications

- ✓ Onsite Healthcare Workshops

- ✓ Programs for Health Care Professionals

- ✓ Speakers Resource Center

Reach out to us at:
Health Options & Alternatives, Inc.
Voice: 866-307-4710
Website: www.healthoa.org
Email: healthoa@att.net